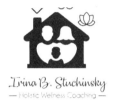

Irina B. Stuchinsky
— Holistic Wellness Coaching —

Healthy Kids
Happy Moms

An Essential Guide for
Moms Raising Healthy Children

Irina B. Stuchinsky

Dedication

I dedicate this book to all the moms who are seeking alternative answers to their kids' health challenges.

Acknowledgments

I want to thank my husband for 15 years of unconditional love, support, and powerful lessons in life and business. I also want to thank my beloved daughters, Isabella and Brianna, who have given me the strength to overcome all the challenges, celebrate the wins, and taught me to listen to my intuition, and to find all the answers within.

I appreciate the unconditional love and lessons my parents and grandparents have taught me to respect others and care for less privileged. A special thanks to all the Institute for Integrative Nutrition (IIN) professors, doctors, and coaches for their guidance and inspiration to live a happy life.

I am grateful for my friend Eleina who showed me alternative ways to convert my home into an eco-friendly place, improve my families health, and start saving the planet… which were things I had wanted to do for a very long time.

Last but not least, a huge thank you to Linda Vettrus-Nichols who helped me finish and publish this book in 30 days and to Steena Marie for a beautiful cover.

Table of Contents

Chapter 1
Nothing is More Important than Our Children

Nine years ago I was overweight, anxious, and depressed. My energy level was at an all time low. I had hormone challenges that ended up keeping me from getting pregnant. I was also in a lot of physical and emotional pain.

I ate highly processed 'junk' food on a daily basis, which made me feel even more miserable than I felt in the morning on an empty stomach. I tried a few popular diets, including Jenny Craig and Weight Watchers. Some of them were effective for a short-period of time, but a few months into them I fell off the wagon and returned to my 'usual' feelings of disappointment and personal failure.

After my husband and I decided it was time to start a family, it took five long years of attempting to get pregnant... to finally get pregnant! We were both shocked to find out that we were having IDENTICAL twins. I did not know how to feel about the news at first, but when it finally hit me that I was going to have not one child but two children, at the same time, I was excited and anxious to go from having no children at the age of 28 (which I thought was old) to becoming a mom of two little ones who would completely depend on me for everything.

When my twins were born, they were preemies. I did everything I knew to keep them healthy and prevent disease: frequent hand washing, clean organic baby food, wiping off toys, cleaning our carpets, and so on. Every time my precious girls got sick with a cold, flu, virus, or stomach ache I got discouraged about the effectiveness of my preventative measures and many times I turned to traditional medicine for answers.

When my girls started daycare, at the age of 2yrs. 6 months, they started to get sick on a regular basis (about every month or two). Every time they got sick I tried harder to 'cure' their illness with what I thought were the answers, like organic foods and hand washing.

As I got more and more concerned about my kids' increasing frequency of colds, viruses, and digestive issues, including stomach aches, nausea, and constipation, as well as newly emerging seasonal allergies and skin irritations, my stress level grew which exacerbated my existing health challenges and created new ones. I was determined to change all of that and I set out on a transformational health discovery journey that would change our lives completely. I started researching and buying homeopathic remedies, but they did not seem to work properly.

Meanwhile I kept hearing from other moms, "Kids have to be sick in order to build up their immune systems so that they don't get sick as adults." That made me furious!! I didn't know how to feel about that. All I knew was that it did not make sense to me. I did let it go because as a new mom I felt I knew very little, compared to moms who had older kids as well as a second or third child.

I tried to figure out why kids in general are often sick and here is what I realized a few years later. Prevention does NOT start when the symptoms are evident. Prevention is an ongoing process that starts before any symptoms of sickness appear and it never stops.

Health is a journey, not a destination!

When I realized 'health is a journey' and I paired that understanding with learning and discovering effective holistic tools and techniques to prevent illness, I started noticing that I did not need to resort to commonly used traditional medications, including a Nebulizer with Albuterol (pure caffeine) and Prednisone, which is a synthetic form of cortisol that can prevent the immune system from doing its job of defending the body against viruses and bacteria if used over a long period of time. I was also using Tylenol, Motrin, antibiotics, and steroids.

The more I learned the more I understood the dangerous effects of long-term use of traditional medications such as organ damage and gut dysbiosis (more bad gut bugs than the good ones) which could potentially contribute to chronic lifestyle diseases, including diabetes, heart disease, and cancer.

Chapter 2
Healthy Kids Are Happy Kids

My twins have been my biggest inspiration to acquire more knowledge in the area of nutrition. About a year ago, I made one of the best decisions in my life. I enrolled in the largest international nutrition and health coaching school in the world. I am so grateful for the knowledge and motivation I've gotten from the most passionate, driven, and happiest people in the world! All of my hard work and dedication definitely paid off.

My girls were constantly sick with recurrent infections, viruses, and digestive issues. I wanted to change our life and become a better informed mom. I eventually went with my gut feeling that 'change was possible'.

Today, as an IIN graduate and a certified integrative nutrition health coach, I am beyond grateful for the exciting year of discovery and two challenging years prior of intense self-learning, dedication, and consistency that brought me to this great chapter in my life. I can proudly say that I was the rock that transformed my own health as well as my kids' health. Your gut knows best, just trust it.

I am now on a mission to share my knowledge and inspiration with other mindful moms who want to take simple steps to optimize their kids' digestion, immune system function, and insulin resistance through the power of nutrition, mindfulness, and healthy habits to prevent their children from developing chronic lifestyle diseases like obesity, cardiovascular disease, and in many cases infertility.

People do NOT need information, there is Google for that. People need support and inspiration to achieve their health goals! Health is not just about what's on your plate. It's about everything else that brings meaning to your life, inspires and fulfills you and therefore, adds years to your life.

Chapter 3
Red Light Foods Green Light Foods

Ever since I can remember, I've been an anxious person trying to be perfect and always striving for the best. My physical health challenges started when I was sixteen years old so my body was sort of set up to fail. I was living a toxic lifestyle.

I had just arrived in this strange, new country, the United States. A country I only knew from Hollywood movies. A trip to Foodtown, Chinese Buffet, and the Dollar Tree, where everything in the store is only one dollar, were my first unforgettable experiences of the abundance, freedom of choice, and endless opportunity. *How could I not get sucked-in* by this lavish lifestyle that I never knew existed?

By the time I became an adult, I was continuing to eat the Standard American Diet (SAD) diet while over using pain medications and antibiotics. I was not getting enough sleep and I was managing my stress by eating at night in front of the TV. After years of self-destruction and slowly depleting my body of essential nutrients, my immune system could no longer fight foreign invaders. As a result, I depended on more and more gut-destroying traditional pain medications, antibiotics, and steroids to fight off inflammation and its negative consequences. I developed a metabolic syndrome, was diagnosed with Hypothyroidism (low thyroid function), and insulin resistance. My hormones were so off that I wasn't able to get pregnant. As you may or may not know, there is this whole biochemical, body connection to getting pregnant.

Our body is so connected. The gut is connected to our brain. It's actually known as the second brain and it helps us to stay in homeostasis, in a balanced state of wellbeing. A healthy gut equals a healthy brain and abundant health.

Living a lifestyle that heals our gut is crucial.

I believe that good health is the foundation, a true building block, for our happiness. Striving for more money to buy a house and obtain more material things isn't what brings happiness. Our health is our wealth!

Wealth doesn't make us happy, health does!

We tend to buy, buy, buy in order to fill the void within. No matter how much we buy we want more and more. Its because material things (objects) don't bring us lasting happiness. When we nourish our bodies with nutritious foods that are full of natural vitamins and minerals, using supplements as needed, laughter and personal connections return to our lives. We find our tribe, develop romantic relationships, create a fulfilling career, and are able to participate in physical activity. We feel complete. Isn't that what life is all about? For me it all boils down to happiness.

Building a house on sand, even if the foundational beams are strong, is going to create a dangerous house to live in.

Healthy nutrition sets a child's body up for success... just like enrolling a child in dance lessons or a particular sport is setting their muscles up for success. The trouble is that without healthy nutrition we set our children up to fail.

Dragging kids off to fifty million after school activities isn't helpful either. Finding one or two activities that your child loves or can learn to love, keeps our children's nervous systems healthy... which in turn allows healthy nutrients to enter their cells.

It's very important to understand that making children do something, especially if they don't want to, creates a disconnect between the two of you. I believe that it's important, as a parent, to inspire them.

When eating a new food, just eat it in front of your kids. Children are curious and love the concept of 'new'. If they ask you what you are eating, tell them the name of the food item and resist saying, "Would you like to try it?" Wait for them to ask you!

Also, showing and sharing something new with your children, that you are trying for the first time... for example a certain yoga pose, allows them to witness you floundering and even failing. This keeps them from thinking that everything they do has to be perfect.

In other words, allow them to watch you face a challenge and see what your reactions are to that challenge. Kids really model us, that's for sure!

You would be surprised what kids will be tempted to try if they see their parents doing it. I am amazed to see the progress my kids have made with the foods that they didn't like and I just figured they would never like them. I would invite them to try different foods I ate and they never wanted to try something new. Then one day I was eating in front of them and they both said "Can I try that?" This kept happening. They just wanted to try something that their mom was eating.

That's why I include mindfulness, in my program. I talk about mindfulness with parents so they can be aware of what they are doing and what they are teaching their children. Kids are watching us all of the time when we don't even realize they are.

I love Dr. Bill Sears' work with the Red Light Foods and Green Light Foods.

He talks about allowing kids to see how they feel after eating something. When it doesn't go real well for them, it's considered a Red Light food. Parents can use a passive tone and say, "Oh, that seems to be more of a Red Light food for you right now."

I teach my kids to be mindful of what they are eating or what they are doing. If they feel uncomfortable or have a feeling that something is out of the norm, I have taught them to let me know. I help them to process what might be going on for them. They seem to need me less and less these days. Isn't that the job of the parent? Allowing your kids to grow up and become less dependent on you?

One morning Isabella was eating cereal and it had milk on it. Right after eating a few bites she said, "Something isn't right with my stomach." It was organic milk with two percent fat content and she was used to that particular brand of milk. However, she was eating a high-quality cereal that she was trying for the first time. Everyone's body is unique, even my IDENTICAL twins are two people with very different food and other preferences, minds, and guts. Even the same person, might at any time, become sensitive to foods to which they were fine eating in the past. The reverse is also possible, kids may be fine eating foods to which they were once sensitive.

Awareness is a great first step!

Note here, what you are aware of right now. Then after you read this book, come back here and note your new awareness and goals for a healthier future for you and your family.

Chapter 4
The Power of Healthy Nutrition

As I mentioned earlier, after years of research and self-discovery, accompanied by skepticism and lack of understanding about nutrition and the power that food has on our vitality and wellbeing, I decided to embark on the educational journey of enlightenment at one of the largest international schools of nutrition and health coaching in the world. This experience has changed my life and my view of the power of nutrition and having a healthy lifestyle forever. It certainly has shifted my priorities and the way I view wellness, happiness, and healthy aging.

Food Cravings

If our body is out of balance we will start having food cravings. For example, when we crave sugary or salty foods, as seen during pregnancy, it is a warning that something is missing from our diet or our life.

We can deconstruct our cravings in order to understand why we have these intense urges. Checking-in and noticing what might be different is very helpful. For example, pregnancy puts a great deal of stress on the body. Magnesium helps us to reduce stress, therefore women who are pregnant tend to experience depleted levels of magnesium. That's where a health coach can come to the rescue because deconstructing cravings can be a difficult process to initially do on your own. We tend to crave foods that release the 'feel good' hormones known as endorphins, produced by our brain and nervous system. They activate the body's opiate receptors triggering a positive feeling in the body and creating the euphoria.

Therefore, if our body, mind, and/or soul are out of balance, for whatever reason, we tend to crave foods that create this feeling of euphoria. Our body is communicating with us in this unique way in order to get our attention. What we don't realize is that there are always healthier options that will produce the same feelings of euphoria, without inflammation that contributes to disease and aging.

People tend to take better care of their cars and their homes. They visit a salon to get their hair and nails done, but forget to take care of their own body. The body never makes mistakes; the heart never misses a beat and lungs never stop breathing. Our bodies are the only mechanism that keeps us alive and well, as long as we take care of them. We can tend to this 'mechanism' and super computer by eating nutritious foods that nourish our bodies and promote healing.

The power of healthy nutrition is endless.

There is a saying, "You don't have a second chance to make a first impression." In a similar way, I would challenge you to think about your life as the only chance you have to make the first impression and you better do it right because there is no second chance.

Reading Labels

Knowing how to read and understand food nutrition labels is crucial for healthy living.

Just a few years ago, I had no idea how to read and understand nutrition labels. As consumers, most of us go to Google, TV, newspapers, magazines, and our physicians for answers about what's good for us in order to stay healthy. I have news for you, what they don't take into consideration is an important concept called 'bio-individuality', sometimes referred to as 'biodiversity'. This means that one person's food is another person's poison. Therefore, no particular diet works for everyone.

Struggling to find answers to my own, as well as my kids', health issues led me to discover the healing power of nourishing, wholesome foods without dangerous refined sugars like corn syrup. I also learned about the neurotoxic effects of artificial flavors and colors like Blue 40 and Yellow 5. Then I learned about the dangers of highly processed and extremely toxic oils known as hydrogenated oils. Partially hydrogenated oils such as corn, soybean, canola, sunflower, safflower, and peanut also play a role in the development of inflammation, an increase in LDL or bad cholesterol, and heart disease. Some of the popular foods containing high amounts of partially hydrogenated oils or partially hydrogenated oils are fries, potato chips, and margarines.

Many of these gut-destroying ingredients, mentioned above, have been scientifically proven to slowly disrupt our immune system function, cause hormonal imbalances, metabolic syndrome, and promote overall inflammation in the body. In the long run, these ingredients create irreversible changes to our cells which in turn can lead to chronic degenerative conditions, including diabetes, heart disease, cancer, and premature aging.

Teaching parents how to read and understand food labels is an integral part of my coaching. My mission is to reduce preventable conditions like constipation, diarrhea, ear/eye infections, and skin issues... using nutrition, mindfulness, and a healthy lifestyle while taking into consideration personalized needs, genetic predisposition, and lifestyle preferences of each individual.

Chapter 5
Prevention is Everything

Yes, prevention is everything. I really, believe in prevention. If you would have asked me four years ago, I would have laughed. I would have told you that prevention doesn't work. Prior to having my twins, I never knew anything about prevention. I never prevented anything! I caused a lot of my health problems.

When I started using prevention strategies, surprisingly I started feeling better and all of a sudden... my kids stopped getting sick as often and as serious as they had when I wasn't mindful about our lifestyle. I was amazed to see this transformation, it really changed our lives and how I look at prevention.

Healthcare is a birthright: You can become an educated consumer and a self-advocate, as well the most powerful voice for your child's well-being and prosperity.

I learned to approach my diet with love and now I know that my food gives me the nourishment I need to be fully me.

After getting junk food out of my house, I switched to eating clean, wholesome, non-GMO foods. Right around that same time, I met a gal in a Facebook group. Her name was Eleina. She seemed different from everyone else. Even though this was a Health group, the others didn't seem to know what they were talking about and didn't have any scientific research to backup their recommendations.

Eleina sounded very concerned and knowledgeable about healthy living and someone who I felt I could trust. I will never forget the day I spoke with her on the phone for the first time. A feeling of hope came over me.

When she introduced me to a U.S. based wellness manufacturer with over 30 years in business and guaranteed the quality of their non-toxic household and other products, I had only one question... "Where had she been all this time?" It was as if she had appeared from nowhere, at the same time that I was trying to figure out how to find NON-TOXIC affordable and effective consumer goods for my household. I really felt like my prayers had finally been answered.

I also thought I was eating healthy until I went to see a functional medicine doctor for the first time. He told me that my diet was healthy according to the U.S. food plate standards, but I needed to add more 'real' protein, like unprocessed meats and healthy saturated fats, including grass-fed butter and extra virgin olive oil. He encouraged me to eat larger portions that could sustain me, without having to eat even healthy snacks between meals.

When a body does not receive proper amounts and certain types of nutrients, this can cause sugar and other bodily imbalances that trigger dangerous systemic reactions that can lead to serious, irreversible damage.

In addition to significant improvements in my health markers, after switching from traditional doctors to a functional medicine doctor, my Hypothyroidism is more controlled with a natural (desiccated) form of Thyroid without any negative effects on my liver, kidneys, and stomach. I also have more energy than ever before.

I'm now a big proponent of prevention and I'm not the only one. It's a huge industry that includes Functional Medicine and Integrative Medicine. There are chiropractors and osteopaths who have prevention built into their practices rather than just acute care.

As part of your own preventive measures for your family, you can begin by slipping great nutrition into spaghetti sauce or something you know your kids will actually eat. For example, if you are using Juice Plus products you know that they deliver key antioxidants and phytonutrients because the company uses a special cold-press technology that preserves all the nutrients. Juice Plus products carry a whole food nutrition label and are not considered supplements. These foods are organically grown. Their products are convenient to use and come in capsules and soft chews.

There is an extensive body of peer-reviewed, third party scientific research (the highest standard of research out there) that has been done on the ingredients within the Juice Plus products.

I found that by adding essential, non-synthetic, plant-based nutrients to my kids' nutrition it didn't take long for their taste buds to change and for my kids to accept healthier options.

Chapter 6
Prevention is an Ongoing Lifestyle

We can transform our health. As I mentioned earlier, my twins were preemies. As toddlers, they kept getting respiratory infections, had dry cough, ear infections and other related symptoms of weakened immune system. My doctor prescribed a nebulizer with steroids including albuterol, which is pure caffeine, prednisone which is a synthetic form of cortisol and can cause multiple metabolic and immune system disturbances with long-term or chronic use, and medications to take daily for dry cough. We had a long road ahead.

You may not get the results that you want and that's okay, try something different.

As a clinician, trained in the traditional pharmacotherapy model, I'm not totally against medications. I want to make it clear, that sometimes we do need antibiotics, sometimes we may need certain medications but in very rare cases and medications are the last resort.

When we have aches and pains there is something going on in the body and it's sending messages to the brain to alert it. Moreover, the brain is called the second 'gut.' A great example of this connection is someone who is anxious and has "butterflies" in the stomach.

Emotional trauma can trigger negative symptoms in the gut and affect gut health. So in addition to having increased risk of brain conditions, such as depression and anxiety, people with past trauma experiences are at a higher risk of developing a gut 'dysbiosis,' a bacterial overgrowth that is very common in the modern world. Gut dysbiosis can also be triggered by an unhealthy diet, causing inflammation in the gut and contributing to a variety of health conditions, including thyroid problems, allergies, and acne. It is estimated that 30 million people in the U.S., predominantly women, suffer from the multiple effects of an imbalance in the gastrointestinal system.

As a psychotherapist, I am trained to focus on the brain. However, my training as an Integrative Nutrition Health Coach prepared me to look at the whole person and embrace each person's uniqueness taking into consideration unique individual genetic makeups, past and present experiences (lifestyle factors), and beliefs. In addition, I am inspired by the science-based approach of functional medicine that addresses the underlying causes of disease instead of just covering up the symptoms and putting a bandaid on them.

There is nothing worse than the bandaid!

We don't need to have aches and pains even in old age. Getting old doesn't mean we have to suffer.

Chapter 7
We Can Transform Our Health

Most approaches to healthy eating dwell on calories, carbohydrates, fats, and proteins. Instead of creating lists of restrictions and good and bad foods, I coach my clients to explore basic improvements and implement gradual changes during our work together. As these pieces accumulate, my clients find that these changes collectively create a much larger impact than they originally anticipated. We work on what they want to improve within the circumstances of their own unique situation.

Health is not about dieting, eating organic or losing weight... it's about leading a fulfilling and sustainable life.

I work with my clients to get in touch with what their body *really* needs because I understand that life happens and I know their needs will change. I equip them with the self-awareness to make the best decisions for themselves in any given circumstance. I believe each person is fully capable of making well-informed decisions. We all have the ability to be our own expert without having to follow the latest magazine article or fad diet.

I empower my clients to define what they value most for their well-being. We use these visions to motivate specific goals that bring them closer to where they choose to be. As their coach, I do not dictate a diet. Together we explore why some foods make them feel better than others and how to strategically use that feedback. Together we co-create their health goals within reasonable time frames and actionable, objective steps so they know exactly what they are working towards.

Here are some concepts that we explore during our work together:

-Eating healthy every day and foods to include in every meal

-Cooking at home

-Drinking lots of water (weight in pounds divided by two) on an average day

-Drinking water instead of sugary drinks or dairy

-Taking daily nature walks

-Half of the plate being fruits and vegetables

-Eating only whole grains (gluten free foods if sensitive to gluten)

-Adding healthy saturated fat (i.e. organic virgin coconut oil, grass-fed butter, ghee, and extra virgin olive oil)

-Including quality protein (i.e. grass-fed/pasture-raised/organic meats, organic cheeses, organic eggs, and low-mercury wild caught fish)

-Cutting out refined carbs (i.e. white bread, white rice, white pasta) and cutting down on carbs in general. Instead eating whole grains and non-starchy vegetables (i.e. asparagus, green beans, brussel sprouts, broccoli, beets, celery, and cauliflower), which are all 'good' carbs.

Here are some of the suggestions I make in regards to helping kids foster healthy eating habits that are simple, fun, and sustainable.

-Encourage your kids to eat 'real', nutritious food

-Educate your children and send clear and consistent messages about the power of good nutrition as well as how healthy habits affect their outer and inner beauty, academic achievements, and the aging process.

-Engage your kids in cooking

-Send home-prepared lunches and healthy, nutritious snacks to school

-Play educational health games with them to inspire healthy choices

-Talk with your kids about information they are getting at school or hearing in the media in regards to dieting, fasting, and creating healthy eating habits

-Role model healthy eating and living habits

Over the past few years, our lives have gradually started to gain a new meaning. We stopped getting sick as often as we did with recurrent infections, viruses, and digestive problems.

Remember that prevention

IS an ongoing lifestyle!

Chapter 8
Long Lasting Results

If we think that we don't have time to incorporate healthy habits into our busy schedules, we deceive ourselves. We can't afford not to, we must take care of ourselves first in order to live a long, vibrant life.

We get to show our children that aging doesn't have to be painful and our genes are not our destiny. In fact, we can change our genes by incorporating healthy lifestyle strategies that have been found to be transformational for our mind, body, and soul.

Malnourished

We don't eat enough nourishing foods for our bodies and then we wonder why we hurt and why we have recurrent infections. When our body is malnourished it can't stay in homeostasis, its losing what it needs.

What is the recommendation for how many fruits and vegetables we should eat per day?

The World Health Organization recommends nine to thirteen servings per day.

That's a lot of food! Quite the investment.

One of the things that I have done is search out a company that has put 'real' food into smaller, power packed increments within capsules and soft chews.

The best company I have found is Juice Plus. I love their philosophy because it supports the World Health Organization's view about fruits and vegetables as an essential part of a healthy diet. Juice Plus helps bridge the gap between when we should eat and what we do eat every day.

The Juice Plus company takes fresh, organically grown fruits, vegetables, seeds, and berries through a special process that does not deplete the nutrient value of those foods. They also put those foods into a capsule or in a chewable for kids. Some adults even prefer the 'chewables' over the capsules.

What I love is how you can take those capsules, open them up, and sprinkle them in the food your child eats. They won't need the whole capsule, the dosage is different for kids. It's a great way to **hide some good nutrition in their food when you start shifting into a healthier lifestyle**.

Juice Plus is the next best thing to fruits and vegetables that can rewire kids' taste buds to enjoy healthy foods and reduce the risk of disease. Parents report reduction in over-the-counter and prescription medications, fewer missed days of school, less visits to the doctor, better health awareness, and improved eating habits after only a year on Juice Plus.

I recommend consuming at least five fruits and five vegetables per day. Adding Juice Plus capsules or 'chewables' to your diet will provide you with plant-based, whole food nutrition from over 30 different fruits, vegetables, and grains.

If the kids are really young, you can even put it in their formula or expressed breast milk. Although if you are breastfeeding, you may not need to do so because you know they will get all of the nutrients they need from the breast milk.

I teach my clients how to be smart about shopping and how to shop on a budget. Their budgets can easily include organic foods because they won't be eating as much. They get more benefits that way. I teach them how to spend less money while eating healthy.

Organic food is power packed and your brain says, "Thank you for feeding me."

People are concerned about organic food being expensive. You only need one organic carrot to ten commercial carrots. Organic isn't more expensive. You are actually wasting your money by not eating organic. Eating organic along with processed foods is super expensive. The processed foods feed your gut bugs which makes you crave more food. At this point, the body is never satisfied and you are making your organs work extra harder… which leads to inflammation, toxic organs, and eventually disease.

When my kids are coming down with a cold or a virus I know I have to heal their gut. I pay very close attention to their gut. They will need more probiotics, the good bacteria that our gut needs in order to replenish itself. Healing starts with the gut.

Dysbiosis in the gut is when there are more bad gut bugs than good gut bugs and that's when we get sick.

When a child is slowing down or a little crabby, that is the best time to take restorative action. In preventive medicine if the nose is drippy your child is in crisis. In the non-allopathic model (mainstream medicine), hospitalization is crisis, certainly not a cold.

I prefer to stay on the other end and stay out of the hospital. I also don't want to get even sicker from the hospital food.

I want people to be more aware and to know what to do first.

I created a cheatsheet that has ten steps you can take to become healthier, to really cleanse your body from toxins. I include ten coaching emails that are delivered after you get the cheatsheet. Each email contains an exercise to help you change your lifestyle for the better. It's a great opportunity for someone who wants to start out with an accountability component. It's like 10 days of free coaching because you can contact me and ask me questions or let me know if you are having any challenges.

You can grab your Free Healthy Kids Junk Food Cleanse Cheatsheet at: www.HealthyKidsCoaching.com

Chapter 9
Being Sick is Not Normal

Just a few years ago, it was common for us to visit our pediatrician every few weeks. This just didn't feel right to me.

I Was Determined to Find Answers

I worked full time and I didn't need anything else on my to do list.

It took me a few years to figure it out, but I found peace of mind and stability in my schedule when I finally gained the confidence and ability to manage my kids health and prevent illness without waiting until they got sick.

Here are a few tips on how to prevent your child from getting sick...

-Diffuse high quality (100% natural) essential oils in your child's room. Lavender oil is the safest for children, but when the child is not in the room diffuse tea tree oil to disinfect the air.

-Every morning, open the windows in your child's bedroom and other rooms if possible, all throughout the year, to get some fresh air into your home.

-IMMEDIATELY STOP using toxic cleaners, laundry detergents/fabric softener sheets, soaps, and other products containing toxic chemicals.

-IMMEDIATELY remove artificial flavors, preservatives, and refined sugar from your child's diet.

Now watch your child's health transform!

I invite you to visit and join my Facebook group

"Healthy Kids, Happy Moms"

https://www.facebook.com/groups/
480093805659010/

Be a part of a great, supportive community of like-minded, health conscious moms and get inspired.

Chapter 10

Purchase Power

As consumers, we tend to be misinformed by the mainstream media, friends, family, and even our own doctors. Therefore, taking charge of our own health and our children's health becomes a crucial part of our survival.

The popular phrase 'knowledge is power', means that as informed consumers we can make healthier food choices.

You don't need to stock up, buying a month of groceries at warehouse stores. The best way to shop on a budget is to pre-plan your meals prior to leaving the house.

Another great strategy to be able to afford quality foods using the same budget is to know how much you can spend on your groceries weekly.

Purifying Your Water

As you may know, fluoride is added to our water supply and toothpastes. This may have undesirable consequences, including hormonal disruption, cognitive problems, weakened immune system function, migraines, and more.

Understanding the effects fluoride has on our bodies is the first step to becoming an informed consumer.

Water Testing for Your Home

You can call your water supplier or use an at-home water test kit to find out if your tap water is fluoridated or not.

Self Advocacy

Self advocacy is crucial to our survival because no one, not even our doctor, knows us better than we do. Moreover, when we become parents we are responsible to advocate for our children and teach them how to be their own advocates as they get older.

Buy Whole Foods Rather Than Processed Foods

Fresh: Buying unpackaged foods makes shopping simple. Packaged foods tend to contain unhealthy, processed and therefore highly inflammatory ingredients.

Clean: Shopping for wholesome, organic produce (when possible) and grass-fed, pasture-raised animal sources can ensure better quality of foods. These are foods high in vital minerals and other nutrients. They are free of toxic pesticides, fertilizers, genetically modified organisms (GMOs), antibiotics, and growth hormones.

Wholesome Foods: Buying wholesome foods can be more efficient and less expensive than shopping for canned or prepackaged foods.

Water: Over 70% of our body consists of water. Thus, water is an essential part of our diet. Clean water is vital for our wellbeing. Most tap water is processed and contains dangerous chemicals, including aluminum, lead, chlorine, fluoride and other unhealthy minerals that can cause hormonal imbalances, infertility, migraines, cognitive decline, and learning problems to name a few.

Buy Local, Sustainable Foods

Buying locally grown and raised food from local farmers helps to support and develop our communities. This will also help to ensure that there will be enough food if our infrastructure crumbles. Another benefit is being able to eat fresher, healthier foods at our local restaurants.

Sustainable foods are produced using farming techniques that support the environment, public health, human communities, and animal welfare.

Consider shopping at local, organic farms.
Organic is one of the first qualities to look for when checking the sustainability of a product. Organic agriculture promotes sustainable soil management, pollinator-friendly crops, and toxin free runoff into nearby waterways.

Two websites that can help you find small local farms in your area are: **www.LocalHarvest.org** and **www.EatWild.com**. Both sites are searchable by zip code.

Shop at Your Local Farmer's Market for Locally-grown, Seasonal Foods

I prefer shopping for seasonal, locally-grown foods rather than buying produce that has been modified through spraying pesticides and herbicides so it can be shipped around the world and sold in big chain grocery stores or supermarkets.

Research shows that supporting our local economy, 'the hands that feed you', is more sustainable, less expensive, and provides better quality produce. You can actually talk to the farmer, learn about their farming methods, and make informed purchasing decisions.

Creating an organic garden may not be for everyone, especially if you are someone like me who does not know how to garden or has made unsuccessful attempts and is looking for a quick and simple way to grow organic fruits and vegetables.

I found an amazing alternative! A Tower Garden from Juice Plus+. It's a great way to share fruits, vegetables, and herbs with your patients/clients, family, friends, and neighbors… and in turn, inspires others to lead healthier lives.

A Tower Garden is a great way to ensure that you are consuming superior quality, fresh foods and actually saving money at the same time. It's simple to maintain, with quick growing, cost effective organic fruits, vegetables, and herbs… in your home or right outside your door.

You don't need to have gardening skills and there is no weeding, tilling, kneeling, or getting dirty in order to maintain this vertical aeroponic system of growing plants in the air and water, without soil. Its compact design makes it possible to fit in a small space and it is an easy way to get the nutrition you need in order to be healthy.

Chapter 11
Supplements

Focusing on food, rather than supplements, is the key to success because supplements cannot substitute or reduce the importance of eating quality food. Once that point is clear, clarifying the role/purpose of supplements is to supplement the nourishing food we are eating. Supplementation is based on the individual needs of a person confirmed through symptoms, lab work, lifestyle, genetics, and environmental factors.

Spend Time in the Sun

I recommend that anyone living in a state like New Jersey or anyone who doesn't have daily access to sunshine, have their Vitamin D levels checked. For those who do get out in the sun, remember the 3-3-3-rule. A third of your skin exposed, three times a week for 30 minutes. This is something I take into consideration when asking my new clients about their lifestyle practices. I find that doing an intake assessment is essential to developing the right plan of care for each client.

Add Spices to Your Cooking

Spices are a great way to supplement your food and can be used to add flavor and aroma. They are well known for their powerful, medicinal cleansing and anti-inflammatory properties.

If you want to give your meals an upgrade... add some new spices to your cooking repertoire. Doing so can make a huge difference in transforming bland meals into flavorful, satisfying dishes.

Chapter 12
My Approach

I practice a holistic approach to health and wellness, which means that I look at how all areas of my client's life are connected.

-Does stress at their job or in their relationship(s) cause them to overeat?

-Does lack of sleep or low energy prevent them from exercising?

As we work together, we look at how all parts of their life affect their health as a whole.

It's rare for anyone to get an hour to explore their wellness goals with a trained professional. As an Integrative Nutrition Health Coach, I create a supportive environment that enables my clients to articulate and achieve their goals. Throughout my education, I have been exposed to the most cutting-edge dietary theories and studied highly effective coaching techniques to help my clients find the right lifestyle that works best for them.

I also guide my clients to find the food and lifestyle choices that best support their child's needs. I help them make gradual, lifelong changes that enable them to prevent their child from getting sick.

I graduated from the Institute for Integrative Nutrition (IIN) where I learned innovative coaching methods, practical lifestyle management techniques, and over 100 dietary theories – Ayurveda, gluten-free, Paleo, raw, vegan, macrobiotics, and everything in between.

I studied with the world's top health and wellness experts including:

Joshua Rosenthal, founder and director of the Institute for Integrative Nutrition

Deepak Chopra, MD, leader in the field of mind-body medicine

David Katz, MD, MPH, director of Yale Universities Prevention Research Center

Walter Willett, MD, DrPH, chair of nutrition at Harvard University

Andrew Weil, MD, director of the Arizona Center for Integrative Medicine

Gabrielle Bernstein, bestselling author and life coach

Susan Blum, MD, MPH, assistant clinical professor at Mount Sinai School of Medicine

Mark Hyman, MD, founder of The UltraWellness Center

Geneen Roth, bestselling author and expert on emotional eating

David Wolfe, raw food leader and nutrition expert

Marion Nestle, PhD, MPH, professor at New York University's Department of Nutrition, Food Studies, and Public Health

Mark Bittman, food writer for The New York Times and bestselling author

Joel Fuhrman, MD, family physician and leading expert on nutritional healing

My education has equipped me with extensive, cutting-edge knowledge in holistic nutrition, health coaching, and prevention of disease. Drawing on my expertise, I work with my clients to help make lifestyle changes and choose health-promoting ways that produce real and lasting results. My clients develop a deeper understanding of food and lifestyle choices that work best for themselves and their child improving their child's daily nutrition, which in turn improves their overall health and happiness.

Through the Institute for Integrative Nutrition (IIN), I also studied a variety of dietary theories and practical lifestyle coaching methods. With my knowledge, I work with my clients to co-create a completely personalized action plan based around their unique goals. These are the goals that will move them towards their ideal vision of being healthier within their own biodiverse bodies, taking into account their lifestyle preferences and the resources they have available to them.

I am also a licensed clinician trained in psychotherapy, with over 10 years of experience in the healthcare system. Health coaching and counseling share major areas of overlap. As a clinician, I have specialized training to assess, diagnose, and work with complex mentally-based conditions. Nobody wants to be sick at any age. However, in the busy, consumer-oriented modern world, we tend to forget about the 'real' role of nutrition and use food to suppress our negative feelings and make us feel satisfied. What many people don't realize is that there are healthier options that have the same positive outcomes on the brain, including dark chocolate and spicy foods.

Childhood trauma can greatly affect our psychological well-being and trigger unhealthy eating patterns. I believe that most adults have had at least one traumatic experience in their lifetime… such as death of a loved one, personal or parental divorce/separation, domestic violence, and/or traumatic brain injury.

I am able to work with complex traumas and I am also able to show my clients the role food plays in their own recovery.

As a coach, I put the power back into the hands of my clients.

Learn more about my training and my unique approach to health coaching at my website and while you are there, **remember to grab your FREE *Healthy Kids Junk Food Cleanse Cheat Sheet***.

Remember that along with the cheat sheet you will get 10 days of free coaching, one instructional email per day. You will also have access to me if you have any questions.

Being healthy doesn't have to be hard.

When was the last time you received the personal attention you deserve
and talked with someone about your health?

Your child's health depends on you.

Additional Information

Myths and Social Perceptions

-It is normal for children to be sick when they start daycare

-Children have to get sick early on in order to build up (boost) their immune system and be able to naturally fight illness

-Being sick as a child helps children be healthier adults

-It is impossible to prevent children from catching viruses/colds/flu when others around them are sick

-Keeping children home until first grade will prevent them from getting exposed to germs early on and protect them from getting sick when they start elementary school

Sustainable Lifestyle Practices

Recycling is a great way to contribute to sustainability of our planet. Most things that we perceive as waste and chose to dispose of can actually be reused if we just put them in a recycling bin.

Upcycling is when you take a used item and create something new with it.

Recycling and Upcycling help to save the planet from unnecessary waste!

Skin

Our skin absorbs everything that we put on it. What we use on our skin is absorbed into the inner layers and into our body. When we are exposed to environmental toxins, such as lead and formaldehyde, which are also found in commonly used items including cosmetics, deodorant, shampoo, and nail polish, we increase our risk of systemic (i.e. endocrine system) toxicity that may cause Autoimmune disorders and cancer.

Childbirth

Growing up in a different culture (Ukraine), I always heard my mom tell me that natural birth was so beneficial for the baby. Even though I didn't understand the exact benefits of vaginal delivery, my mind was set and I was determined to deliver without a C-section. I knew that with twin pregnancy there was a higher risk for an emergency C-section, but that was the only reason for the operation in my "dictionary." As a clinician, I understand that it's important to consider the risks when medical decisions are made. In my mind, simply having a twin pregnancy does not make it a medical necessity for having a C-section. I am the proof of that even though my doctor, family, and friends had other ideas.

Breastfeeding

Breastfeeding is essential for a baby's healthy development because of the essential nutrients, vitamins, and minerals in the breast milk. Formulas, on the other hand are full of artificial ingredients and therefore need to be selected and administered with caution. When babies are on a formula, they must be closely monitored by their caregiver in order to spot early signs and symptoms of formula sensitivities.

Pasteurized and Homogenized Milk

The same is true for when pasteurized and homogenized milk is introduced. It is pointless and can even be dangerous to give homogenized milk to a baby because of the toxins that are formed in the milk during homogenization.

Importance of Dental Hygiene Habits

The mouth is the largest opening to the whole body. As a new parent, I've overlooked the importance of practicing regular dental hygiene beyond just a regular brushing twice per day. After conducting more research, graduating from the IIN, and discovering that one of my twins had cavities and an infection that caused us to extract one of her molars, I quickly realized the importance of 'appropriate' and consistent brushing habits.

Tongue Scraping

One such habit is tongue cleaning (also known as scraping). Flossing also plays a significant role in sustained internal health. Who wouldn't like to avoid cavities or dental infections? Knowing 'how' and knowing that many things/conditions are preventable is part of living a healthy lifestyle.

Toothbrush Replacement

It is important to regularly replace ones toothbrush and to soak it in hydrogen peroxide. If there has been an illness in the home, make sure to replace all of the toothbrushes especially after infections or the flu.

'Bad Gut Bug' killers & Probiotics (Foods & Supplements)

-Fermented foods such as milk kefir, watermelon, beets, homemade sour pickles (see recipe below), kombucha, purple or regular sauerkraut, and kimchi

-Juice Plus fruit and vegetable capsules (can also be sprinkled in baby formula or on baby food and foods for the whole family)

-Raw Probiotics for Kids (powder) by Garden of Life (children 3 months and older)

-Nature's Answer, Sambucus Kid's Formula for children (ages 4 and older)

-Dr. Formulated Probiotics Organic Kids (chewables) by Garden of Life (ages 4 and older)

-Little Warrior *Children's Immunity Blend* by Khroma (www.khromahearbs.com)

-Vitamin D-3 liquid formula by WholeFoods (ages 4 and older)

Meditations

Simple Meditations

Sit in a comfortable position with your feet on the ground

Close your eyes

Breathe

- Take a few deep breaths (inhale with your nose, hold your breath for a few seconds and exhale through your mouth)
- Repeat a few times
- While taking deep breaths, envision an ideal place that brings peace and tranquility to your mind and helps you to relax
- Turn on ocean waves sounds, birds singing, or wind blowing (optional)

You can also go to your mobile phone application store and download guided meditations and mindfulness meditations.

Intake Questions & Recipes

What are your child's favorite foods?

What does your child like to do for fun?

Has your child ever witnessed or experienced a traumatic event (i.e. death of a loved one, parental divorce, domestic violence, being bullied, traumatic brain injury)?

What is your child's favorite sport or activity?

When it comes to your child's health, what are your goals?

Recipes

Homemade fermented (sour) dill pickles:

Sterilize your jar and the lids in a 'water bath' (boiled water) and let it cool to room temperature

Put grape leaves on the bottom of the jar

Cut long quarters of cucumbers and pack them tightly in the glass jar

Add dill stems and flowers

Pack cloves of garlic, a few on the bottom and a few on the top

To make the brine:

Add 3 cups of water

Add 2 cups of organic (5% acidity) white vinegar

Add ¼ cup of pickling salt (non-iodized sea salt or kosher salt) and bring it to a boil

Pour the brine into the jar to cover the cucumbers

Wipe the top rim with a clean paper towel and put the sterilized seal and the ring on top of the jar to seal it tightly

Put the jar in a hot water bath for 10-15 min.

Keep the pickle jars in a cool dark place, sealed for at least 24-48 hours and on up to 4-6 weeks

Yogurt cake: Preheat oven to 350 degrees Fahrenheit

Use a Springform Pan

Lightly grease your pan with grass-fed butter or oil or line the pan with parchment paper

Dry Bowl-Combine
1 ¼ cup/165gm sprouted whole wheat flour/coconut or almond flour
1/4 cup/30g ground almonds (optional for flavor)
1 tsp=4 gm baking powder

1/2 tsp=2 grams baking soda
1/2 tsp=2 grams sea salt or pink Himalayan salt

Flavor the cake with organic lemon or orange zest (grate the yellow or orange skin using a micro grater)

Whisk everything together

Wet Bowl-Combine
2 large organic eggs
3 quarters=180g of plain, whole fat organic yogurt
½ cup of extra virgin olive oil (flavorless)
1 tsp/4 grams pure vanilla extract
1 cup/200 grams of organic cane sugar or stevia
Mix the dry and the wet ingredients together with a whisk

Add berries, plums, peaches and/or dark chocolate chips (optional)

Put the batter in your Springform Pan and place in the oven

Bake for 35-40 min
-Rotate the cake front and back after the first 20 min.
-Insert a toothpick to check if it's ready

Blueberry muffins: Preheat oven to 375 degrees Fahrenheit

12 cup Muffin Tin

Lightly butter or use paper liners

Wet Bowl-Combine

1 large egg (organic)
1 cup of whole fat unpasteurized organic plain yogurt
1/3 of a cup (30 ml) of flavorless extra virgin olive oil
1 tsp of pure vanilla extract

Dry Bowl-Combine

3 cups of coconut, almond, or gluten-free flour
1/2 of a tsp of organic cane sugar or stevia
1/4 tsp of baking powder
1/2 tsp of baking soda
1/4 tsp of Himalayan pink salt or sea salt
1 or 1 and ½ cup of organic blueberries or berries of your choice (if you use frozen, don't thaw them)

Mix wet and dry ingredients together and gently stir until the batter is thick
Add a zest of organic lemon/orange (optional)

Fill muffin cups with the batter to the top

Bake for 15-20 minutes until the muffins turn brown.

Insert a toothpick in the center of a muffin to check if it's ready

Books I Recommend

"Eat Fat, Get Thin" by Mark Hyman, MD.

"Grain Brain: The Surprising Truth about Wheat, Carbs, and Sugar-Your Brain's Silent Killers" by David Perlmutter, MD with Kristin Loberg.

"Nutrition and Inflammation" by Dr. Gary Fettke.

"Successful Aging" Second Edition by Mary O'Brient, MD

"The Dental Diet" by Steven Lin, MD.

"The Whole Foods Diet: The Lifesaving Plan For Health And Longevity" by John Mackey, Alona Pulde, MD, Matthew Lederman, MD.

"Your Bodies Many Cries for Water" by Dr. Batmanghelidj, M.D

"Prescription for Nutritional Healing: A Practical A-to-Z Reference to Drug-Free Remedies Using Vitamins, Minerals, Herbs & Food Supplements" Fifth Edition, by Phyllis A. Balch, C.N.C.

With seven million copies sold, Prescription for Nutritional Healing is the nation's number one-bestselling guide to holistic health. For more than twenty years, people have relied on this invaluable reference as a guide to improving health through nutrition and supplementation. Now thoroughly updated, the fourth edition incorporated the most recent information on the benefits of alternative healing and preventive therapies.

Whether you are looking for relief from a particular ailment or simply wish to maintain optimum health, this book quickly and easily provides an abundance of information to design a complete nutritional program.

Phyllis A. Balch, CNC, was a leading nutritional counselor for more than two decades. Convinced that nutrition was, in many cases, the answer to regaining and maintaining health, Balch testified before Congress on the power of natural healing.

About the Author

As a woman who struggled for five years to get pregnant and ended up with premature twins, who continually got sick, Irina B. Stuchinsky did tons of research. She is a licensed clinician trained in psychotherapy, with over 10 years of experience in the healthcare system. Irina also holds a coaching certificate from the Institute for Integrative Nutrition. She saves her clients time and money by passing on her knowledge so they have the energy to deal with raising a family. Irina believes that health is not about dieting, eating organic or losing weight, it's about leading a fulfilling and sustainable life.

CPSIA information can be obtained
at www.ICGtesting.com
Printed in the USA
LVHW010312150819
627732LV00006B/162/P